# HOMEOPATHY UNVEILED

# HOMEOPATHY
# UNVEILED

## AN EXPLANATION OF
## HOW IT REALLY WORKS

*WRITTEN AND ILLUSTRATED*

*BY*

*GIRI WESCOTT*
*R.S.HOM. (NORTH AMERICA)*
*B.R.C.P. (HOM.)*

HOMEOPATHY UNVEILED
AN EXPLANATION OF HOW IT REALLY WORKS
Copyright © 1994 by Giri Wescott
ISBN 0-9641323-1-1
Library of Congress Catalog Number
95-092159

Published by
Satyam Publishing
832 School St. #5
Napa, Ca.
94559

This  book is in no way
meant as a guide for self prescribing.

Printed in the U.S.A.

# CONTENTS

Illustrations....vii

Acknowledgments....xi

Introduction....1

Principles of
Homeopathic Medicine....7

What is Homeopathy....11

Susceptibility and Vital Force....13

Law of Similars....17

Energetic Medicine....19

Primary and Secondary Action....23

Cure or Suppress....27

Obstacles and Antidotes....29

Preventive Treatment....39

Patient Expectations....41

Watch Your Symptoms....43

Conclusion....47

Glossary....51

Notes....59

Bibliography....61

About the author....63

# ILLUSTRATIONS

The illustrations in this book depict some of the sources
from which Homeopathic medicines are derived.

Agaricus Muscarius....viii

Chelidonium Majus....x

Citrullus Colocynthis....xiii

Samuel Hahnemann....xiv

Naja Tripudians....9

Drosera Rotundifolia....10

Lycosa Tarentula....12

Leontodum Taraxacum....16

Sepia Officinalis....21

Strychnos Nux Vomica....22

Iris Versicolor....26

Paris Quadrifolia....28

Euphorbium Officinarum....38

Cyclamen Europeum....40

Bryonia Alba....46

Asarum Europeum....50

Magnolia Virginiana....58

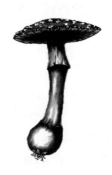

**AGARICUS MUSCARIUS**

This book is dedicated to
Sri Satya Sai Baba.
With love and gratitude.

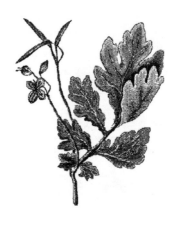

**CHELIDONIUM MAJUS**

## ACKNOWLEDGMENTS

I would like to express my thanks to those who have helped me produce this little work. First, I owe my deepest gratitude to my wife, Pari. Through all the years of hardship, her unfailing support and love made it possible for me to fulfill my aspiration to study homeopathy.

Next I would like to thank my teacher S. C., without whom I would still be groping in the dark. She gave generously of her time. She invited me into her work, for which I will always be grateful. I would also like to thank innumerable friends for their encouragement, support, and help. Each one played an indispensable role in bringing my dreams to fruition. Among these, special mention must be made of Mel and Shubi Raymond, who welcomed my wife and me into their home during the years I studied in England. Their generosity and hospitality will never be forgotten. Mel also spent many hours working on the original layout and designed the cover.

Thanks also to Mary Racine who donated her valuable time to help edit the text, to Bob Tajima for the many hours of work he put into typesetting and to Karl Robinson M.D. for his valuable editorial advice. Dr. Robinson as well as Dr. Richard Moskowitz have helped me in various ways throughout the years, for which I would like to offer my sincere thanks.

My thanks also to Murray Feldman R.S.H., Durr Elmore D.C. N.D. and Iain Marrs who took the time out of their busy lives to review the book.

It is my sincere hope that the information contained herein will help to clear some of the clouds of mystery and confusion surrounding the art and science of homeopathic medicine.

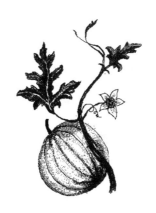

**C**ITRULLUS **C**OLOCYNTHIS

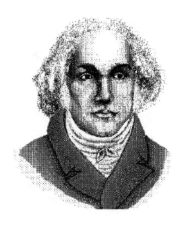

Samuel Hahnemann

# INTRODUCTION

## A BRIEF BIOGRAPHY OF SAMUEL HAHNEMANN

The founder of the therapeutic system known as homeopathy was Samuel Hahnemann, born in 1755 in what is now Germany. Hahnemann was a genius of his time and a great humanitarian. From an early age his accomplishments in many different fields were astonishing. He was a master of eight languages and by the age of twelve he was already renowned as a teacher of Greek.

Well known by his contemporaries as a great physician, Hahnemann possessed an intricate knowledge of every branch of medical science. He was also known as one of the great analytical chemists of his time. His discoveries in this field (the black oxide of mercury and tests for the purity of wine), were still in use into the early twentieth century.

In 1792, he was one of the earliest pioneers of the humane treatment of those suffering from mental illness, at a time when the customary procedure was to cage and torture the patient.

Hahnemann was also an accomplished writer, publishing more than 116 major works during his lifetime. Among his writings on many topics are what may be considered the first articles on air pollution (1792-1795), as well as a commentary on the role of hygiene in the prevention of contagious illnesses. Hahnemann was respected even by his detractors as a man highly educated in pharmacy, botany, astronomy, geology, and physics.

The medicine of Hahnemann's time was based on the assumption that disease was caused by excesses of the four humors. These excesses had to be expelled by any means. Medical "developments" based on this assumption produced methods of treatment such as venesection, cautery, and the use of deadly poisons like mercury, all very harmful to the patient. Hahnemann became a forceful voice of protest against these methods, which he felt were brutal, inhumane, unnatural and responsible for killing and crippling more patients than they helped. His ideas were revolutionary, even by modern standards. He insisted that disease and health were due to various states of the patient's vital resistance and that, to cure any disease, the physician must cooperate with and encourage this resistance and certainly do nothing to injure or suppress it.

Hahnemann's first writings on homeopathy appeared in the year 1796 in an article entitled "The New Principle for Ascertaining the Curative Powers of Drugs". In the major works on homeopathy that followed, such as *The Organon of Rational Medicine* (1810), *The Chronic Diseases and Their Peculiar Nature* (1828) and *The Materia Medica Pura* (1811), he expounded on the principles of homeopathy.

In his long practice (nearly fifty years) of the science that he formulated, Hahnemann remained steadfastly devoted to the relief of suffering as his motivating force. He never charged the poor for treatment and he never accepted payment unless the patient was cured.

Hahnemann died in 1843 at the age of eighty-eight. By this time, his original work on homeopathy, the *Organon,* had gone through five editions, the sixth being published posthumously, each edition was revised in light of his most recent discoveries. It should be noted that his writings were always based on his extensive observations of the responses of the human body to drugs, contagious influences and chronic diseases, rather than on hypothesis or opinion. Hahnemann clearly indicated when he was expressing an opinion that had not been verified by his experiments and observations.

*"The truth of the homeopathic healing art has found so much acceptance from physicians far and near, that it can no longer be obscured, and still less extinguished. . . . I rejoice at the benefit it has already conferred on humanity, and look forward with intense pleasure to the not distant time when, though I shall be no longer here, a future generation of mankind will do justice to this gift of a gracious God, and will thankfully avail themselves of the blessed means He has provided for the alleviation of their bodily and mental sufferings".*

*Samuel Hahnemann*
*Organon*
*Preface, 3rd Edition*
*1824*

*The material in this book is derived mainly from Samuel Hahnemann's writings, in an attempt to explain the science of homeopathy in a concise fashion to all those who are interested in this subject .*

# THE PRINCIPLES OF HOMEOPATHIC MEDICINE

"Thus homeopathy is a perfectly simple system of medicine remaining always fixed in its principles and in its practice". Samuel Hahnemann, Introduction, *Organon,* 5th Edition

"Homeopathy asserts that there are principles which govern the practice of medicine". James T. Kent, Lecture 1, *Lectures on Homeopathic Philosophy*

## 1. Vital Force

"Animates the material organism in health and in disease". (Org. para. 10)

## 2. Susceptibility

"The inimical forces, . . . to which our. . . existence is exposed, . . . do not possess the power of morbidly deranging the health of man unconditionally: but we are made ill by them only when our organism is sufficiently disposed and susceptible". (Org. para. 31)

### 3. Similars:

"The curative power of medicines, therefore, depends on their symptoms similar to the disease but superior to it in strength". (Org. para. 27)

### 4. Provings

"Pure experiments on the healthy for the purpose of ascertaining their real effects and powers, in order to obtain an accurate knowledge of them". (Org. para. 120)

### 5. Succussion

"The homeopathic system of medicine develops the inner medicinal powers of crude substances by means of a peculiar process unique to homeopathy". (Org. para. 269)

### 6. One Remedy at a time

"In no case is it requisite to administer more than one single, simple medicinal substance at a time". (Org. para. 272)

### 7. Direction of Cure

"It is evident that man's vital force. . .adopts a plan

of developing a local malady on some external part, solely for this object, that by making and keeping in a diseased state this part which is not indispensable to human life, it may thereby silence the internal disease". (Org. para. 201)

## 8. Miasms

"The only real fundamental cause and producer of all the other numerous, I may say innumerable forms of disease. . .". (Org. para. 80)

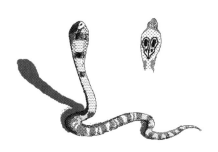

**NAJA TRIPUDIANS**

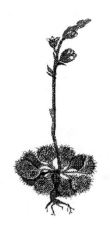

DROSERA ROTUNDIFOLIA

## WHAT IS HOMEOPATHY?

Homeopathy is a healing system based upon the principle of the "Law of Similars." (*"Homeo"* meaning similar and *"pathy"* meaning suffering). Homeopathy asserts that the curative relationship between medicine and patient is one of similarity between the patient's symptom picture and the symptoms specific to the remedy. This principle is directly obverse to traditional systems of medicine, which are "antipathic" or "allopathic", which mean against or different from. The following text provides an overview of the application of the Law of Similars.

The most important element in the practice of homeopathy is *individual susceptibility.* Single symptoms or the symptoms of a single organ system are not the disease, but rather only partial expressions of the total state of the organism. Traditional medical doctors tend to specialize, treating different organ systems separately. The homeopath treats the person as a whole, perceiving all of the symptoms as different aspects of one total condition.

*Disease is not an entity* therefore medicines have no power to destroy this supposed *entity.* The allopathic concept is that an invading organism is responsible for a great many forms of disease. Modern medicine is built around this way of thinking about disease. The homeopath relates all forms of disease back to the individual state of susceptibility.

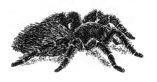

LYCOSA TARENTULA

## SUSCEPTIBILITY AND VITAL FORCE

Homeopaths understand disease to be a state of inherited or acquired *susceptibility* of the *vital force* within each living being. Without this state of susceptibility, contagions will not "take" in any individual. Even the most virulent strains of contagion are not universally contagious; an individual must be susceptible. Susceptibility will determine how and when a given individual is affected by even the most deadly poisons or viruses. In theory, allopathic medical philosophy agrees with this position, except for the assumption of the existence of a "vital force," which cannot be seen. Although allopathic medicine may agree in theory, one individual's susceptibility is generally not a factor in the practical application of modern medicine. However, in the application of homeopathic medicine, it is the key.

When considering the existence of a vital

force, it is essential to understand that all matter is actually energy. Matter is controlled by the forces of energy within it, yet no energy is actually seen. This is a truth proven by modern physics. Energy is known by its force and influence over matter: the subtle but powerful force which controls the movement of the planets cannot be seen, yet we know it exists by the influence it has on solid bodies that we can see. The force within a magnet cannot be seen, yet we are aware of its presence by its power to attract iron to itself. There are numerous other examples.

A corpse cannot move its limbs, cannot think or speak, or resist the tendency of all organic matter to decompose into its simplest constituent elements. This demonstrates the presence of a force or energy responsible for life. From the homeopathic perspective, it is this dynamic force within us that controls all functions, material substances and structures of the body, from the most subtle to the most dense. Therefore, health and disease are defined by the state of the vital force and its effects on the body and mind of the individual.

In homeopathic terms, if the vital force is in "order," "balance," or "homeostasis," the sensations, functions and structure of the organism are in order. When we are well, we are not aware of our heart pumping, our food digesting, our blood flowing. . . and so on. However, when we are "unwell," in a state of disease, we experience many abnormal sensations and functions. In prolonged chronic disease, this altered or disordered state results in tissue changes, such as tumors and ulceration. Disease is defined as a "deviation from the former healthy state," a deviation from the state in which we felt relative comfort, well-being, and the absence of symptoms.

*Susceptibility* is the basis of this deviation. Why does one individual "catch" a contagion and another, exposed to the same environment, not "catch" it? The answer is that we all have a different state of susceptibility. We are not all susceptible to the same circumstances at the same time, in the same way. At one time, we may be susceptible, at another time not. This demonstrates that the vital force is a dynamic rather than a static force. It is constantly adapting, adjusting and fluctuating according to circumstances. When our individual state of susceptibility comes into contact with just the right circumstances, symptoms are produced by the altered vital force. The vital force is responsible for all sensations and functions of the body, including these symptoms. When it is in "balance," we are in a state of health in all our sensations and functions. When, due to susceptibility, the vital force cannot adjust appropriately to outer circumstances, we experience symptoms. Susceptibility is the cause of disease. Homeopathy treats this cause as opposed to treating the effects of susceptibility, that is, the symptoms.

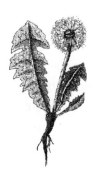

LEONTODUM TARAXACUM

## LAW OF SIMILARS

Homeopathy regards symptoms as the outward expression of the inner vital force. They demonstrate the inner natural susceptibility or the individual's "weakest points." According to the Law of Similars, it is through the language of symptoms that the organism calls for the substance which it needs to restore itself to equilibrium. All substances have a specific relationship to the human body in terms of the symptoms they produce. Any toxic substance will alter the human organism in a unique way, altering the sensations and functions throughout the body. No two substances produce exactly the same symptoms, however similar they may seem.

As stated previously, the Law of Similars is *the* curative relationship between patient and drug. A substance must be identified that in its toxic state, produces symptoms similar to those of the patient (similar in sensation, location, functions, factors of aggravation and amelioration, and other features). The totality of the essential symptoms of both patient and remedy must match, so that the medicine, given in its non-toxic, homeopathic form, truly affects the patient's total susceptibility.

In homeopathic practice, single symptoms are never taken to represent the whole. A patient is not the knee, nose, or head. Homeopaths never prescribe one medicine for this symptom and one medicine for that. There is only *one* vital force and therefore, only one state at a time to be treated. That particular state is treated as a whole, from the innermost qualities of mind and emotions to the outermost sensations and symptoms of the body. When a medicine is prescribed according to the similarity to the total symptom complex, the vital force responds, being touched at all its "weakest points." It is as if the remedy enters a "window of susceptibility."

## ENERGETIC MEDICINE

The ideas introduced in the preceding sections such as susceptibility, vital force, homeostasis and disease as a state rather than an entity, are guiding tenents in homeopathic philosophy. Therefore, we must continue this "energetic" train of thought. Health is essentially an energetic state of fluctuating balance, constantly changing and adapting to circumstances. Disease is defined as this same energetic state, which has been altered by abnormal susceptibility to particular circumstances. It is this abnormal susceptibility which causes the organism to produce symptoms. It follows that only energy can cause this state to return to its previous condition of fluctuating balance or homeostasis.

To the homeopath, all matter is actually energy. Yet energy, which is in potential form in all matter, must be liberated for use in medicine. Homeopathic medicines are made from animal, vegetable, and mineral substances, and are prepared according to the Homeopathic Pharmacopoeia of the United States. The method of preparation is a process of dilution and succusion (kinetic agitation) in serial repetitions to produce subtle remedies of great power. This appears to be a contradiction in terms. However, though the remedy is very subtle, it is very powerful due to the individual susceptibility of the patient for whom it is specifically prescribed. According to the Law of Similars, this subtle remedial force is prescribed according to the similarity between the symptoms that a substance (in its unprepared natural state) can produce in the healthy human and the symptoms of the patient. When remedial agents are prescribed by following this natural Law of Similars, the remedy enters the patient's "window of susceptibility." The patient will respond to very little of the remedy—the very least possible is the homeopathic guideline.

The homeopathically chosen remedy, acts as a catalyst effecting changes in the vital force. It acts like a spark causing the vital force to return to the state of equilibrium that characterized it in health. Symptoms disappear because they have no life of their own. They are caused by the disordered state of the vital force due to abnormal susceptibility. Once that has been removed, the vital force is set in order, causing symptoms to disappear.

A homeopathic remedy does not actually cure the patient. Only the inherent, indwelling vital force, which is responsible for the creation and maintenance of the organism, can accomplish this. Remedial agents can only trigger that force to move into a state of proper, fluctuating balance wherein this natural curative function can occur.

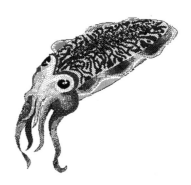

**Sepia Officinalis**

21

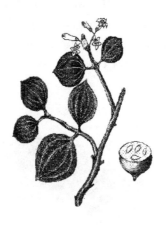

**STRYCHNOS NUX VOMICA**

## Primary and Secondary Action

How homeopathic remedies work is a mystery to most people. Even patients who have relied on the homeopathic system for their health care for years have little understanding of what actually takes place. A brief explanation may resolve some questions.

A given individual's response to any substance is determined, in large measure, by his or her particular susceptibility and the strength of the dose. Generally there will be similarities in the responses of different people. For example, coffee usually has two effects on those who drink it. Initially, one feels the enlivening of spirits and energy which is the primary reason for its use. However, as time goes on and the effects of the caffeine wear off, there is a depressing action causing the user to feel tired, limp, and dull. These two phases of the drug action are called the primary and secondary actions respectively.

This double action is not only seen in the use of caffeine. It is also observed in the use of all other drugs. In general, the secondary action of the drug is roughly equal in strength and opposite to the primary action. The primary effects are the vital force's "passive response" to the influence of the drug (based on the individual's susceptibility), while the secondary action is the rebound or "active response" of the vital force, attempting to "free itself" from the drug influence. In homeopathic science, this natural phenomenon is utilized to trigger a curative movement in the vital force.

The homeopathic procedure involves prescribing a remedy that matches the patient's symptom complex. The medicine is given in a highly dilute and dynamic energetic form. This infinitesimally small dose may cause a slight, almost imperceptible aggravation of the presenting symptoms because of the remedy's similarity to the disease symptoms. Its influence is slightly stronger than the natural disease. Due to the remedy's subtlety, its action is quickly spent and easily overcome by the vital force. A gentle rebound or secondary action then takes place. This secondary action, which is opposite and equal in strength to the primary action, causes the vital force to exert only enough energy to free itself from the momentary influence of the remedy thereby moving gently toward a state of equilibrium. This differs greatly from the uncomfortable and sometimes dangerous rebound that occurs with toxic, suppressive medicines.

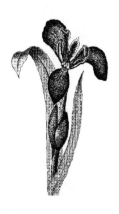

IRIS VERSICOLOR

## CURE OR SUPPRESS

From the homeopathic perspective, all disease states that a person experiences throughout life are interrelated actions of the vital force due to inherited influences. In the course of successful treatment, as one state is thrown off by the vital force, the previously suppressed state emerges. So there arises a succession of previous states in reverse chronological order, an indication to homeopaths that they are curing rather than merely suppressing.

This reappearance of previous states does not emerge all at once, nor does the patient have to experience all of the suffering of previous states. Often the experience is like passing milestones with symptoms of the past flitting by. The patient recognizes a symptom that hasn't been felt in "so many years." As present states disappear and previous states arise, well-being returns. The object is not just the removal of discomfort and pain. The patient's level of energy should increase, the mental and emotional states become brighter; all the signs of true health become tangible experiences.

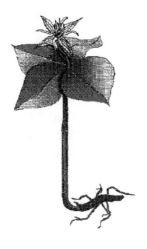

**PARIS QUADRIFOLIA**

## OBSTACLES AND ANTIDOTES

When pursuing homeopathic treatment to address acute or chronic conditions, the patient must rethink many long-held beliefs and habits. It is a great challenge for many to understand that it is the vital force alone which is responsible for, and capable of healing the body, often without any interference. Therefore, one of the greatest obstacles to homeopathic treatment is the patient's inability to understand the need to eliminate the habitual use of suppressive measures to treat symptoms.

All over-the-counter or prescription drugs and even "natural" remedies (herbs, etc.) must be avoided for acute problems as well as for individual chronic symptoms. Such substances tend to erode the overall health of the patient due to their suppressive action. The vital force carries on all of its functions in an orderly manner, including the exteriorizing of symptoms from the interior when the vital force has met contagion.

This exteriorized symptom picture is actually a very orderly arrangement in its totality. Therefore, symptoms should not be altered or tampered with by taking any therapeutic substance, whether "natural" or pharmaceutical, which does not address the total state of the individual. The entire state must be considered as the natural, harmonious expression of the inner condition of susceptibility and then treated in its entirety by applying the Law of Similars, as described earlier.

Patients who use allopathic medicine(s) daily for a serious chronic condition should consult their homeopath, so that treatment may be tailored to the special needs of the case. Ultimately, the long-term plan will be to assist the patient in gradually and safely abandoning the drug, whenever possible, while supporting the patient with the indicated homeopathic remedy. No long-term curative benefits can be expected as long as the patient is taking daily doses of any toxic substance.

It is important to explain the effects of using birth control pills and recreational drugs. Any toxic substance taken on a regular basis produces symp-

toms which are known as iatrogenic or drug induced. These symptoms, while being artificial elements in the case, also suppress other natural
symptoms which may have been important guiding features of the natural chronic case. This creates a serious obstacle to curative success.

Suppression takes place because the drug-in-
duced symptoms are dissimilar to the symptoms of
the natural disease. To paraphrase Hahnemann's
*Organon,* when two diseases (or symptoms) meet
in the same individual, the stronger disease or
symptom suspends the weaker. When the stronger
has exhausted itself, the weaker emerges uncured.
In context, the symptoms induced by birth control
pills and other drugs are stronger than the disease
symptoms due to the frequent toxic dosing.

As said before, *there is only one vital force and
this manifests any internal disorder outwardly.*
The drug's influence on the vital force becomes ir-
resistible with frequently repeated doses. Repeti-
tion creates an artificial susceptibility or artificial
drug disease. The vital force is compelled to manifest this artificial susceptibility or disease. As it
does so, the natural susceptibility and its symptoms are suspended and suppressed, since the vital force can only manifest one generalized disease

condition at a time. As long as the patient continues using the drug, the natural disease symptoms are kept down. Because the natural susceptibility can no longer be exteriorized, relieving the internal influence of disease, natural susceptibility gets worse over time. Stronger and stronger doses of the medicine must be taken. In some conditions it may be very dangerous for the patient to discontinue use of the drug due to this aggravated state rearing its head in a violent and sometimes fatal return of the suppressed natural disease. (See Primary and Secondary Action.)

Strong coffee or tea, narcotics (including sleeping pills), amphetamines (including weight loss pills), hallucinogens, marijuana, alcohol, and/or cigarettes are some of the most commonly used drugs. While it is understood that some of these habitually used substances cannot be stopped overnight, it is essential that the patient have a sincere commitment to abandoning their use as soon as possible.

In regard to birth control pills and IUDs, it should be noted that the menstrual cycle is a very fundamental function. Serious consequences on the general state of well-being cannot be avoided when natural physiology is manipulated in such a manner. Therefore, nothing permanent can be gained from any therapeutic treatment if a woman continues to use such methods.

The issue of antidoting homeopathic remedies by eating certain foods is often misunderstood. In general, remedies cannot be antidoted in this way. Remedies are not material substances. The remedy is not a substance in the blood performing any particular function in the body to react to another ingested substance. Remedies are dynamic energetic catalysts. They generally cannot be antidoted by the use of a material substance.

Once the remedy touches the patient's tongue, its job is complete; its force is spent. If the remedy was correctly chosen according to the patient's symptom picture, his or her vital state of susceptibility feels this catalyst and changes begin taking place in the vital force. This evolving state of the vital force produces the changes that are evident to the patient. This state cannot be "antidoted," except by a substance which has a similar symptom picture. Therefore, only another dynamic substance can "antidote" a previous one.

It is widely assumed and misunderstood that caffeine and various other substances have a universal antidotal action on homeopathic remedies. Hahnemann states:

> Considering the minuteness of the doses necessary and proper in homeopathic treatment, we can easily understand that during the treatment everything must be removed from the diet and regimen which can have any medicinal action, in order that the small doses may not be overwhelmed and extinguished or disturbed by any foreign medicinal irritant.[1]

In his book, *Chronic Diseases and Their Peculiar Nature,* he explains further:

> As to diet and mode of living I shall only mention a few remarks, . . . in order to make the cure possible, the homeopathic practitioner must yield to circumstances in his prescriptions as to diet and mode of living, and in so doing, he will much more surely, and therefore more completely, reach the aim of healing, than by an obstinate insistence on strict rules which in many cases cannot be obeyed. . . Moderation in all things, even in harmless ones, is the chief duty of chronic patients.[2]

Hahnemann's friend and student C.M.F. Von Boenninghausen writes in his *Lesser Writings:*

It is plain that every article of food ought to be free from medicinal virtue, since this causes variations in the patient's condition, and thus must make healthy men more or less ill, even if this should be only transitory . . . Even more important in this direction is the observation frequently made, that as a rule only such medicinal substances act in a disturbing manner, on substances given before as have homeopathic relation to it, i.e., which have the virtue and tendency of producing similar effects on healthy persons. On this alone the antidotal action rests which a number of medicines show, and by this may be explained how it comes, that many an otherwise antidotal substance passes by without causing any disturbance. . . The potencies which are at this day carried higher . . . have so much increased the intensity of the medicinal virtue that all grossly material influences can affect it but little or not at all.[3]

Also, according to The great American Homeopath, James Tyler Kent,

"... Diet lists and lists of things the patient should avoid belong to the routinist. The only ironclad rule that you must work under in all cases is, be sure the remedy is similar, and then see that the foods agree".[4]

Therefore, it is clear that any disturbing effect a

food substance may have on the reaction the vital force has produced after the administration of a curative remedy is due only to that food's ability to produce a medicinal action in the susceptible individual.

Toxic substances of any kind can cloud the symptom image in the chronic case or create an entirely artificial image which overlays the natural chronic one. Treatment then becomes impossible because of the confusion of symptoms and ongoing poisoning of the individual. "Antidoting" is not a major problem. Any mention of it in the writings of the great classical homeopaths is in the following context.

Homeopathic treatment emphasizes individuality. If a patient has a susceptibility to a particular substance and if the susceptibility is sensitive enough and the influence of the substances great enough, a temporary, acute reaction may be produced. This acute state may "antidote," or to use Hahnemann's words, "overwhelm and extinguish" the action of the previous dynamic remedy, as the acute state is dissimilar to it in terms of its symptom picture. Therefore, the chronic state is temporarily suppressed. (See Primary and Secondary Action pg 23) This is similar to the suppressive action

36

of an acute illness. An acute self-limiting disease, when present, suppresses the chronic state until the acute state completes its natural course. It should be noted, however, that in any chronic state there are certain parameters within which the dynamic, fluctuating vital force may move, without leaving the chronic state.

When the vital force returns to the expression of the chronic state, it is as if a constitutional remedy were never given, and the chronic symptoms which were temporarily suppressed by the acute state then arise. At this point, the chronic remedy is repeated in order to carry on the chronic treatment uninterruptedly. This is the case with all acute, self-limiting symptom manifestations, whether triggered by contagion or by allergen. Acute pain, fright, grief or toxic substances can cause a similar reaction. All are capable of producing an "extinguishing" action if the susceptibility is great enough and the influence strong enough.

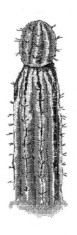

**EUPHORBIUM  OFFICINARUM**

## PREVENTIVE TREATMENT

The homeopathic view of health and disease can be summed up by the following simple equation: Inheritance + Circumstances = Present State. In therapeutics we have no control over circumstances, but homeopathy can produce changes in the inherited influences which are the source of all presenting or future symptoms. By changing one of the factors in the equation we change the outcome.

If the inherited influences in patients can be quieted the ground will be prepared for a healthier human species generally. This is because each parent passes on to their offspring the state of susceptibility that he or she is in at the time of the conception. If each successive generation is treated homeopathically, the family will progressively get healthier and healthier in terms of reduced sensitivity to contagion and the circumstances which trigger chronic diseases from within. This will ultimately lead to the greater well-being of the human race itself.

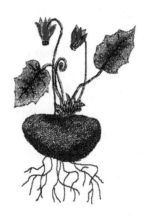

**CYCLAMEN EUROPAEUM**

## Patient Expectations

Homeopathy aims at nothing less than quieting acquired and inherited disease influences. This takes time to accomplish. The final resolution of chronic health problems does not happen overnight. However, as soon as the correct remedy is identified and prescribed, the patient often experiences changes almost immediately. A disease condition took years to create and it must be systematically unraveled. Not all symptoms disappear at once, and the patient must communicate often with the practitioner via telephone and follow-up consultations. When acute conditions such as colds, flu, infections and injuries occur, it is essential that the patient contact the homeopath. They are part of the ongoing process of the case and will be treated, if necessary, with remedies compatible with the constitutional treatment. Whatever symptoms come and go in the course of treatment, the patient should experience an overall increase in energy and stamina and a sense of mental and emotional well-being.

The homeopath, as well as the patient, must always remember that whatever the name of the disease, whatever its supposed cause, vital susceptibility is the true cause and to remove this susceptibility is the only real cure. By keeping the focus on the general state instead of individual symptoms permenant  cure is most efficiently accomplished.

Because the homeopath treats the underlying predisposition any type of state, regardless of the traditional diagnosis, may be benefited by an on-going course of homeopathic treatment. Some of the essential ingredients to curative success are rapport, which is absolutely necessary so that honesty and clearity of expression may exist, as well as patience and commitment. When the working partnership of the homeopath and client possess these qualities curative benefit is a likely outcome.

# WATCHING YOUR SYMPTOMS

To prescribe for any case homeopathically, very detailed information is essential. It is therefore of the utmost importance for patients to observe themselves carefully until the individualizing features are collected. If one desires homeopathic treatment, one should become as fluent in the proper narration of symptoms as possible. This helps the homeopath gather the information that will point to the appropriate remedy.

The following is a brief guide to the information patients should learn to observe and report whenever consulting with their homeopath.

## SYMPTOMS TO NOTICE

### 1. Modalities

Notice the time of the day and circumstances when you are better or worse. Do this with each particular complaint as well. It is a good practice to try cold or hot compresses on areas of pain to see which one feels best. Also try pressure and rubbing.

## 2. Sensations

Wherever a sensation or pain occurs, give an exact description and location, (such as, "burning on the left side of my throat"). Also give the "modality." (See #1).

## 3. Discharges

Notice discharges carefully as to color, consistency, odor if any and any other peculiar feature; such as acrid, ropy, or bloody.

## 4. Thirst and hunger

This pertains to natural thirst, not forced fluid intake. What do you desire to eat or drink? What aversions do you have, if any, and why? Do you desire cold or hot drinks and why?

## 5. Perspiration

This is very important to be aware of on waking and at other times. Notice if it occurs at various places such as the head, hands, feet, back and chest or if it is general. If it is cold or hot. Take note of any unusual odors.

## 6. General state

Are you restless or lethargic, chilly and wishing to remain covered or hot and wanting to be uncovered? Are you hypersensitive to external stimuli?

## 7. Mental state

Learn to report your mental/emotional characteristics in the clearest, most spontaneous fashion. After years of psychological counseling, patients often begin to describe themselves with the jargon of the therapist. This can be a very real obstacle to the homeopath's clear understanding of a person's true personality as seen in the light of natural behavior.

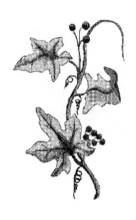

**BRYONIA ALBA**

# CONCLUSION

Nearly 200 years have passed since the first publication of Samuel Hahnemann's Organon. Throughout the long history of this amazingly gentle and curative system misunderstanding has obstructed its permenant acceptance in American society. Now with the slow awakening of vitalistic consciousness and with the discoveries of modern physics the day is dawning that will grant homeopathy the permenant place that it deserves as an indispensible healing system for suffering humanity.

In our time we are witnessing an unparalled appearance of new disease states throughout the worlds population. For many, the old therapeutic answers to these tormenting conditions are no longer sufficient. People everywhere are seeking for new answers and  more and more of them around the world are finding Homeopathic medicine as the solution to their personal health problems.

With its sound and proven principles Homeopathy offers to us all a system of healing based on natural law. It is a curative as well as preventative system badly needed in our time wherein the patient is a participant in the healing process rather than merely a recipient of often suppressive and invasive practices. Homeopathy reminds us that health, disease and cure are all based upon vital susceptibility and that the responsibility of all practitioners and patients alike is to safegaurd and cooperate with this healthy vital susceptibility at all times. It reminds us that we are all the caretakers of our own health and that we can not manipulate the forces and functions of the body in the name of medicine, or to conform to fads and convenience, without paying a heavy price.

We must all remember that the human body is a wonderfully delicate and balanced ecosystem. True health is achieved only by the respectful consideration of the vital force governing this system and the natural functions and symptoms established therein. It must be understood that these symptoms are the vital forces own efforts to achieve and maintain optimum health and fulfillment in response to the innumerable stresses of life. Its is by learning to understand the language of symptoms and how they guide to the curative treatment that the patient and practitioner together become a powerful team for the renewal of health and personal fulfillment of the individual and therefore, in time, of society itself.

Homeopathy stands ready and invites the scrutiny of all sincere inquiry so that the misunderstanding of the past may be dissolved and the sick may be cured.

## *Aude Supere*

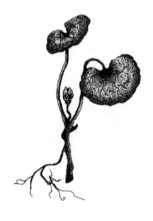

**ASARUM EUROPEUM**

# GLOSSARY OF HOMEOPATHIC TERMS

## Acute disease
Any disease state not directly related to the chronic state in its symptoms. A self-limiting condition characterized by a period of onset (see prodomal), climax, and resolution. Contagious disease state or one caused by contaminated food or water. A temporary state caused by unusual circumstances which create a symptom picture unlike the chronic state.

## Aggravation, homeopathic
Temporary excerbation of the presenting symptoms of the patient after taking a homeopathic remedy. The exteriorization of previously suppressed states (see section on primary and secondary action).

## Allergen
Any substance to which the individual has a peculiar sensitivity.

## Allopathy

The traditional orthodox medical system. Any therapeutic approach that prescribes medicines which produce symptoms different from those the patient experiences in his or her natural disease state. Any therapeutic approach which treats individual symptoms and/or does not recognize the existence of the vital force.

## Antidote

Any substance which counteracts the action of a previously ingested substance. Any homeopathic remedy which can cause the curative action of a previously prescribed remedy to cease. Any circumstance which is severe enough, or to which the patient is sufficiently sensitive, to cause the vital force to backslide into the previous disease state after responding to a curative remedy.

## Antipathic

Any therapeutic approach that prescribes drugs which produce symptoms opposite to those of the patient's natural disease.

## Catalyst

The remedial influence which initiates and precipitates a process of change or adjustment in the vital force, especially without being involved in or changed by the consequences.

## Chronic Disease

Any condition marked by long duration and/or frequent periodic exacerbation which has no prodromal period and which continues to worsen with time.

## Contagion

Any communicable disease causing agent.

## Continuum

That quality of the vital force that is characterized by its continuous exteriorization from the subtle to the gross, from mind to body, from innermost to outermost.

## Cure

"The rapid, gentle, permanent restoration of health" in mind and body. "The removal and annihilation of the disease in its whole extent."[5]

## Dynamic

Continual productive, energetic activity and force.

## Equilibrium

The dynamic state of adjustment and balance between the opposing forces of external and internal nature, i.e. circumstances and the patient's susceptibility.

**Exteriorization**

The vital force's ability to manifest symptoms from within. "The outwardly reflected picture of the internal essence of disease."[6]

**Hahnemann, Samuel**

The founder of the homeopathic system (1755-1843).

**Hering's Law**

The observed pattern of exteriorization of the vital force as it manifests disease symptoms and as the curative response develops after the administration of the remedy. The pattern of resolution in acute diseases. From within the interior of the vital force and body, manifesting outward; from the upper part of the body, downward; from more important organs to less important ones; resolution of symptoms in reverse chronological order from their development.

**Health**

That state wherein "the reason gifted mind can freely employ this living healthy instrument for the higher purposes of our existence."[7]

**Homeostasis**

Continual balance and equilibrium.

**Iatrogenic**

Drug-produced symptoms.

**Inheritance**

The subtle energetic influences passed on from one generation to the next.

**Miasm**

Inherited predispositions to produce particular forms of disease. The three miasmatic influences identified by Hahnemann are; Psora, Syphilis, and Sycosis.

**Modality**

That which modifies a specific pain or symptom making it better or worse.

**Organon**

Hahnemann's original writings on the science of homeopathy.

**Pharmacopoeia**

The official authority and recognised standard for the description of drugs and their preparation.

**Potency**

The degree of dilution and agitation a homeopathic remedy has gone through in preparation. Three standard scales exist. The decimal (1/10), centesimal (1/100), and LM (1/50,000).

## Primary action

The vital force's (passive) action of manifesting the effect of any medicinal agent. Iatrogenic disease symptoms or artificial drug disease. After the administration of a homeopathic remedy this primary action sometimes causes a slight temporary aggravation of the presenting symptoms.

## Prodromal period

The period of onset of acute illness.

## Provings

Double-blind experiments on healthy humans for the discovery of the effects of drugs on the human body and mind.

## Secondary action

The vital force's action of recovering its previous natural state after being altered by a medicinal substance.

## Similars, Law of

The curative relationship between the patient's total symptom image and the symptoms produced by the therapeutic agent as seen in the provings (See provings).

**Succusion**
The kinetic agitation in the process of homeopathic remedy production.

**Suppression**
Any therapeutic alleviation of symptoms which does not begin in the internal general state and which does not cause an exteriorization of previous disease states leading to the removal of abnormal susceptibility.

**Susceptibility**
That attribute of the vital force characterized by continual fluctuation and adaptation to external circumstances in order to achieve and maintain equilibrium. Susceptibility governs all the responses of the individual to all external stimuli.

**Symptom Complex**
The individual's total group of symptoms including those on the mental, emotional, and physical levels.

**Totality**
The group of individualizing symptoms from the symptom complex which indicate the curative remedy in any particular disease state.

**Vital Force**
That animating force of life which is responsible for

all the characteristics of health and for all the manifestations of disease.

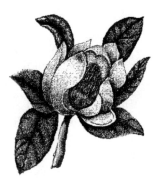

**MAGNOLIA VIRGINIANA**

# NOTES

1. Samuel Hahnemann, *Organon,* (New Delhi: B. Jain Publishers, 1991), paras. 259-260.

2. Hahnemann, *Chronic Diseases and their Peculiar Nature* (New Delhi: B. Jain Publishers, 1980), pp. 197, 112.

3. C. M. F.Von Boenninghausen, *The Lesser Writings,* (New Delhi: B. Jain Publishers, 1979) pp. 270.

4. James Tyler Kent, Minor Writings (New Delhi: B. Jain Publishers, 1988) pp. 390

5. Hahnemann, *Organon,* para 2

6. Ibid., para. 7

7. Ibid., para. 9

# BIBLIOGRAPHY

Close, S. 1981. *The Genius of Homeopathy.* New Delhi: B. Jain Publishers.

Cook, T. 1981. *Samuel Hahnemann, The Founder of Homeopathic Medicine.* Northamptonshire, Great Britain: Thorsons Publishers Ltd.

Haehl, R. M.D. 1922. *Samuel Hahnemann, his life and work.* New Delhi: Jain Publishers.

Hahnemann, S. 1980. *Chronic Diseases and their Peculiar Nature.* New Delhi: B. Jain Publishers.

_____. 1980. *Lesser Writings.* New Delhi: B. Jain Publishers.

_____. 1991. *Organon. 6th ed.* New Delhi: B. Jain Publishers.

Kent, J.T. 1981. *Lectures on Homeopathic Philosophy.* Berkeley: North Atlantic Books.

_____. 1988. *Minor Writings.* New Delhi: B. Jain Publishers.

Roberts, H. 1992. *Principles and Art of Cure by Homeopathy*. New Delhi, B. Jain Publishers.

Von Boenninghausen, C.M.F. 1979. *The Lesser Writings*. New Delhi: B. Jain Publishers.

Weir, Sir J. *Samuel Hahnemann and his Influence on Medical Thought*.

## ABOUT THE AUTHOR

Giri Wescott has studied homeopathy since 1980 while working in Calcutta, India at a home for destitute children. There he began an intense comparative study of Hahnemann's Organon and James Tyler Kent's Lectures on Homeopathic Philosophy.

On returning to the west he studied with an important British homeopath from 1986-1988. He has taught at London College of Homeopathy, Manchester College of Classical Homeopathy and the Farnham Royal College of Homeopathy in England.

Mr. Wescott now conducts his practice in Napa California.

If you would like to be on our mailing list or if your group or organization would like lectures or seminars by Mr. Wescott on introductory or advanced homeopathy please write to:

Giri Wescott
C/O Satyam Publishing
832 School St.#5
Napa, Ca.
94559

# Order Form

### To Order Homeopathy Unveiled
### directly from the publisher;

Company Name:_____

Name:_____

Address:_____

City:_____State:_____ Zip:_____

Quantity____Price_____

Tax (CA. Residents Only)_____

Shipping and Handling_____

Grand Total_____

Send your check or money order to:
Satyam Publishing 832 School St. #5, Napa, CA. 94559

**Retail Price:** $9.00

**Sales tax:**

Please add 7.25% for books shipped to California addresses.

**Shipping and Handling:**

$2.50 for the first book & $.75 for each additional book. Surface Mail may take up to 4 weeks.